One Point Acupressure for Insomnia

Acupressure Therapy to Fall Asleep Fatser and Overcoming Sleeping Disorders

Dan Phillips PhD

~DEDICATION~

~1~

~LARRY~

For your unwavering support, encouragement, and friendship. Your presence in my life has been a constant source of inspiration. Thank you for your invaluable kindness and belief in my journey. This book is a token of appreciation for your enduring friendship and steadfast encouragement.

TABLE OF CONTENT

CHAPTER 1

Understanding Insomnia and Sleep Disorders: This chapter provides an overview of insomnia and different sleep disorders, their causes, and the role of acupressure in managing them.

One of the most important biological functions for preserving general health and wellbeing is sleep. But for a lot of people, the peace that comes with a good night's sleep is still unattainable because of a variety of sleep problems, the most common of which is insomnia. This chapter explores the complex realm of sleep disorders, illuminating the various difficulties they present and exposing readers to the possibility of using acupressure as a comprehensive method of treating these problems.

The Sleep Problem

Known as the "sleep thief," insomnia is a common sleep problem that impacts millions of people globally. It is typified by trouble getting to sleep, remaining asleep, or having non-restorative sleep. People who struggle with insomnia are caught in a never-ending cycle of exhaustion, agitation, and diminished cognitive abilities. However, insomnia is not a single disorder; it can take many various forms, ranging from brief sleeplessness brought on by stress or a shift in schedule to chronic insomnia that lasts for weeks or even months.

A Spectrum of Sleep Disorders Beyond Insomnia

Even though insomnia is one of the most well-known sleep disorders, a number of other sleep-related issues also take center stage. There is a spectrum of sleep disorders that includes sleep apnea, parasomnias including sleepwalking and night terrors, narcolepsy, and restless leg syndrome. Each condition has its own set of symptoms and underlying reasons. For example, sleep apnea causes respiratory problems that disrupt sleep, leading to sleep disturbances and extreme daytime sleepiness. Comprehending various diseases is essential, since a holistic approach to sleep health needs to take into account their unique characteristics.

Examining the Root Causes

In order to treat sleep problems, it is necessary to first identify the complex network of underlying causes that leads to their emergence. The sleep-wake cycle is frequently disturbed by lifestyle variables such excessive caffeine intake, inconsistent sleep schedules, poor sleep hygiene, and elevated stress levels. In addition, underlying medical disorders including anxiety, depression, and chronic pain can exacerbate sleep difficulties. Further aggravating sleep difficulties is the widespread use of technology and the continuous connectedness it provides, which can interfere with the body's circadian rhythm.

The Significance of Acupressure for Sound Sleep

Acupuncture and other traditional healing methods have gained a lot of interest again as people look for non-invasive, holistic treatments for sleep issues. The foundation of acupressure, which has its roots in traditional Chinese medicine, is the idea that the body's meridians carry vital energy, or "qi." A disruption in this flow can result in a number of health issues, including trouble sleeping. Acupressure seeks to reestablish the harmonious flow of qi by applying targeted pressure to particular acupoints along these meridians, thus fostering a state of balance and harmony.

Acupressure's Promise

By treating the underlying imbalances that lead to sleep disturbances, acupressure offers a special method for improving sleep health. Important acupoints are stimulated in order to trigger the body's self-healing mechanisms, which aid in stress relief, anxiety reduction, and relaxation—all of which are essential elements of restful sleep. Acupressure is also a desirable option for people looking for natural substitutes for pharmacological interventions due to its non-invasive nature.

We'll go into more detail about acupressure and its potential to treat insomnia and other sleep disorders in the upcoming chapters. Through the integration of contemporary scientific knowledge with the knowledge of traditional Chinese medicine, our goal is to provide readers useful tools and insights to enhance their general health and quality of sleep. As we set out on this trip, it's critical to keep in mind that there are many different ways to achieve peaceful sleep, and acupressure is a useful tool in this endeavor.

CHAPTER 2

The Basics of Acupressure Therapy: Introduce readers to the fundamentals of acupressure, explaining key pressure points and their relevance to promoting better sleep and overcoming insomnia.

The value of getting a good night's sleep in a world where digital connectivity and nonstop activity are the norm cannot be emphasized. However, many people are unable to achieve the elusive state of deep, restful sleep, which can result in a variety of health problems and a lower quality of life. In the quest for restorative sleep, acupressure, an age-old technique, provides a comprehensive method of treating sleep-related issues. The principles of acupressure therapy are explored in detail in Chapter 2, along with the importance of certain pressure points in promoting better sleep and treating insomnia.

Exposing Acupressure Treatment

An ancient Chinese therapeutic method called acupressure is based on the idea that the body's meridians, or channels, are where essential life force, or "Qi," is believed to circulate. An imbalance or blockage of this energy can cause a number of physical and mental illnesses, including insomnia. By applying pressure to particular places along these meridians, acupressure seeks to restore the balance of Qi and support the body's natural healing capacities.

The Science of Pressure Point Development

The idea of pressure points, or certain locations on the body with higher concentrations of Qi and connections to different organs and systems, is fundamental to the practice of acupressure. It is thought that applying focused pressure to certain areas will stimulate them, releasing tension, enhancing circulation, and reestablishing energy flow.

Because it induces the release of endorphins and encourages relaxation, acupressure may be a useful tool in the fight for better sleep.

Important Pressure Points for Improved Sleep

Number One: Yintang (the Third Eye Point):

The Yintang point, which is between the eyebrows, is thought to help with stress relief and mental calmness. Light pressure applied to this spot can help reduce anxiety and create a calm, sleep-inducing environment.

2. Spirit Gate (Shenmen):
Shenmen point, located on the ear, is associated with the heart and mind. In order to achieve emotional balance and ease restlessness, stimulating this region is necessary for a restful night's sleep.

3. Anmian (Slumber with Calm):
The Anmian point, which sits behind the ear, is particularly linked to problems with sleep. It's

well known for promoting serenity and helping people get rid of sleeplessness.

4. Spirit Gate, Heart 7:

This pressure point, which sits on the wrist, is thought to help calm the mind and reduce worry. Additionally linked to heart health, it enhances general wellbeing and improves the quality of sleep.

5. Spleen 6 (Intersection of Three Yin):

This point, which is located on the inner leg, around four finger-widths above the ankle, is well known for its function in controlling the neurological and digestive systems. Acupressure can assist in reducing gastrointestinal pain that could interfere with sleep by focusing on Spleen 6.

Using Acupressure to Help Beat Sleeplessness

A common sleep problem called insomnia, which is defined by trouble falling or staying asleep, can have a serious negative effect on a person's physical and emotional well-being. In order to treat insomnia, acupressure addresses its underlying causes in a non-invasive, drug-free manner.

Stress Reduction: Insomnia is frequently brought on by prolonged stress. Because acupressure relieves tension and encourages relaxation, it can lower stress levels and create a more sleep-friendly atmosphere. Stress reduction can be greatly aided by pressure points that target anxiety and emotional imbalance, such as Yintang and Shenmen.

Controlling Sleep Cycles: Insomnia can result from disturbances in the circadian rhythm, which is the body's internal clock. Acupressure seeks to balance the body's natural sleep-wake cycle by applying pressure to points related to the neurological system, such as Heart 7 and Spleen 6.

Increasing Melatonin Production: A restful night's sleep depends on the hormone melanatonin, which controls sleep. Acupressure's ability to induce relaxation and lower stress levels supports the body's natural melatonin synthesis, which facilitates easier falling asleep.

Increasing Blood Circulation: The body needs healthy blood circulation to carry nutrients and oxygen throughout it. Acupressure enhances blood flow to the brain by activating pressure points such as Anmian, which fosters the peaceful, tranquil state of mind required to initiate sleep.

Accepting Acupressure: A Comprehensive Approach to Healthy Sleep

Modern lifestyles continue to make it difficult to get restorative sleep, but acupressure shows up as a comprehensive and tried-and-true remedy. Instead of just treating the symptoms, acupressure therapy targets the underlying causes of sleep disturbances by opening up the body's natural energy channels and clearing obstructions. Acupressure combined with a nightly regimen might provide a mild and efficient way to get rid of insomnia.

Final Thoughts

The basic ideas of acupressure therapy and its potential for improving sleep quality and curing insomnia have been clarified in Chapter 2. Readers are given the knowledge necessary to take the first steps toward better sleep quality by knowing the science underlying pressure points and how they relate to different body systems. Bridging the gap between traditional knowledge and contemporary research, acupressure provides a complete and all-natural answer to the common desire for restorative sleep. Acupressure beckons as a route worth taking in the pursuit of improved sleep, enabling people to discover the restorative potential found within their own bodies and minds.

CHAPTER 3

One Point Acupressure Technique: Focus on the specific acupressure point(s) that are particularly effective for inducing sleep and improving sleep quality. Describe the technique, pressure application, and recommended routines.

Within the field of acupressure, there is one location—a gateway, if you will—that can open the doors to peaceful sleep and revitalizing rest. This chapter takes readers on a path toward better sleep and overall well-being by focusing on this essential acupressure point and the methods that can be used to harness its power.

The Passage to Peace: Examining the Acupoint that Promotes Sleep

Tucked away within the complex system of energy meridians is the acupoint called "Shenmen," which translates to "Spirit Gate" in English. This acupoint, which is situated on the crease of the wrist, represents the meaning of its name by acting as a bridge between the outside world and the inner peaceful world. Shenmen, also known as Heart 7 or HT7 in scientific circles, is well known for its ability to reduce anxiety, calm the mind, and create a deeply relaxed state that is ideal for sleeping.

The Method Disclosed: Using Acupressure on Shenmen

In order to fully utilize Shenmen's sleep-promoting properties, acupressure, an age-old technique, must be used. Start by finding a peaceful, distraction-free area where you may sit comfortably. Reach out with your arm extended, palm up, and find the spot on your wrist where your hand and arm connect. The Shenmen acupoint can be found by lightly running your fingertips down this crease until you feel a tiny depression there.

Apply firm pressure to this acupoint gradually using your thumb or index finger. While maintaining enough gentleness to prevent pain, the pressure should be just right to activate the point. Apply steady pressure in gentle, rhythmic circular motions for a duration of one to two minutes. While doing so, pay attention to your breathing, letting each inhalation and exhalation lead you to a more relaxed condition.

Opening the Portal: Suggested Acupressure Techniques

Pre-Bedtime Ritual: Include acupressure from Shenmen in your regimen before bed. Before going to bed, use the method on each wrist for two minutes. To maximize the relaxing effect, use this with deep breathing techniques.

2. Midnight Reset: Apply Shenmen acupressure in a dimly lit space if you awaken in the middle of the night and find it difficult to go back to sleep. This helps to relax the mind and makes it easier to fall back asleep quickly.

3. Daily Stress Relief: Use acupressure as part of your regular routine to reduce stress and improve the quality of your sleep in general. To stimulate Shenmen and

help release tension and keep your mind in equilibrium, find a quiet time of day.

4. Mindful Wind-Down: Establish a calm ritual to wind down by stretching lightly, applying Shenmen acupressure, and lowering the lights. Incorporate this with a cup of herbal tea and some relaxing music to let your body know it's almost time for bed.

A Word of Caution: Although acupressure is generally safe and well-tolerated, it's crucial to speak with a healthcare provider before starting any new wellness regimen, particularly if you are expecting or have underlying medical concerns.

By creating a space where calm sleep can thrive, integrating the One Point Acupressure Technique into your daily routine creates a link between traditional medicine and contemporary understanding. As you begin your acupressure adventure, keep in mind that being conscious and consistent are essential. You create the conditions for deep sleep at night and reviving energy in the mornings by gently pressing the tips of your fingers together.

CHAPTER 4

The Science Behind Acupressure for Sleep: Explore the scientific research and studies that support the efficacy of acupressure in addressing insomnia. Explain the physiological mechanisms involved in acupressure's impact on the sleep-wake cycle.

The search for good sleep has grown more difficult in the midst of the never-ending activity of contemporary life. For those who struggle with insomnia and other sleep issues, acupressure is an age-old technique that presents a viable means of regaining peaceful sleep. Here, we explore the scientific literature and experiments that demonstrate the effectiveness of acupressure in treating insomnia and reveal the physiological processes underlying its effects on sleep-wake cycles.

Linking Western Science with Traditional Knowledge

The effectiveness of acupressure is not limited to anecdotal evidence and conventional wisdom, despite its historical roots. An increasing number of scientific studies have been conducted in an attempt to solve the puzzles around this behavior and how it affects sleep cycles. Numerous research studies have looked at how acupressure affects different parts of sleep, providing insight into the physiological changes that take place in the body both during and after acupressure treatments.

Neuronal Control and Stress Mitigation

Acupressure's effect on sleep is mostly due to its capacity to affect the neurological system. Studies reveal that activation of particular pressure sites causes neurotransmitters like endorphins and serotonin to be released. These substances have the ability to promote emotions of wellbeing and relaxation, which successfully lowers tension and anxiety, which are frequently the causes of sleep disorders.

Moreover, research using neuroimaging methods has demonstrated that acupressure can alter brain activity, especially in regions linked to emotion control and sleep-wake cycles. Acupuncture's general soothing impact is enhanced by the activation of these regions, which facilitates a state that is favorable to falling asleep.

Regulation of Circadian Rhythms

The sleep-wake cycle is controlled by the circadian rhythm, which is the body's internal clock. This rhythm's disruptions may result in sleeplessness and other sleep-related issues. The effects of acupressure on the control of the circadian rhythm have been well researched. Notably, after receiving acupressure treatments, researchers have noticed variations in melatonin synthesis.

Often called the "sleep hormone," melatonin is an essential hormone that tells the body when it's time to go to sleep. Research has indicated that acupressure might increase the generation of melatonin, which may facilitate sleep and help people stick to a regular sleep schedule.

Balance of the Autonomic Nervous System

The autonomic nerve system (ANS) regulates blood pressure, digestion, and heart rate, among other involuntary body processes. Sleep patterns can be disturbed by

ANS imbalances. Research on the effects of acupressure on the autonomic nervous system (ANS) has shown that certain pressure points can activate the parasympathetic branch of the ANS, which is in charge of encouraging rest and relaxation.

For example, studies have shown a correlation between increased parasympathetic activity and decreased sympathetic nervous system activity (the "fight or flight" response) when the Shenmen pressure point on the ear is stimulated. This change toward a more relaxed state adds to acupressure's overall calming effects and increases the possibility that they will improve the quality of your sleep.

Oxygenation and Blood Circulation

Good blood flow is necessary to supply oxygen and nutrients to the body's systems, including the brain. Studies that have monitored changes in blood flow after acupressure sessions have shown how acupressure affects blood circulation. Acupressure works by applying pressure to particular places on the body to improve circulation. This helps to make sure that the brain and other essential organs get enough oxygen.

Increased blood flow helps to promote mental clarity, which is necessary to start sleep. The Anmian pressure point, which is situated behind the ear, is especially linked to improving blood flow to the brain, which promotes a calm and comfortable frame of mind that is ideal for sleeping.

Final Thoughts

The investigation of acupressure's effects on sleep by science presents an intriguing synthesis of traditional knowledge and contemporary insight. The physiological principles underlying acupressure's effectiveness in treating insomnia and fostering better sleep have been clarified through research. Acupressure facilitates deep and restful sleep by altering blood circulation, the autonomic nervous system, circadian rhythm, and brain control.

Research on the complex relationships between acupressure, the body's energy pathways, and sleep is leading to a more thorough comprehension of the potential benefits of this age-old technique. The connection between traditional wisdom and contemporary scientific research is becoming more and more apparent with each new study that illuminates the physiological alterations that take place during acupressure treatments, offering people a comprehensive method for curing insomnia and promoting a restorative sleep cycle.

CHAPTER 5

Creating a Personalized Acupressure Routine: Guide readers on how to design a tailored acupressure routine based on their specific sleep patterns, individual needs, and any underlying health conditions.

In the world of acupressure, there is no one-size-fits-all method for achieving peaceful sleep. An individualized strategy is needed to maximize the benefits of acupressure for better sleep quality, as every person has different needs, sleep patterns, and underlying health issues. This chapter will act as a manual to help you create a customized acupressure practice that will meet your unique needs and lead to restorative sleep.

First Step: Self-Awareness and Evaluation

Take the first step toward developing a customized acupressure program by starting a self-discovery journey. Think for a moment about your sleep habits and difficulties. Do you have trouble going to sleep, remaining asleep, or both? Are you having trouble sleeping because of any particular triggers, such worry, anxiety, or discomfort? An method that is specifically tailored to you starts with an understanding of your own sleep landscape.

After that, think about any underlying medical issues you might have. Do you have depression, chronic pain, or any other health conditions that could affect how well you sleep? Recognizing these elements is essential because they will influence the acupressure sites and methods you decide to use.

Mapping Your Acupressure Points is Step Two.

Now that you have a better understanding of yourself, it's time to identify the acupressure points that will form the foundation of your unique regimen. For example, if anxiety significantly interferes with your ability to sleep, think about points like Shenmen (HT7) for mental clarity and Neiguan (PC6) for relaxation. If your nights are ruined by physical pain, use Zusanli (ST36) to release stress and improve your general state of relaxation.

Furthermore, keep an open mind and consider topics not covered in the book's earlier chapters. Look up information on acupressure and traditional Chinese medicine online, or get advice from a trained professional to find spots that speak to your particular requirements.

Step 3: Customizing Methods to Your Requirements

Once your acupressure spots have been determined, work with the methods that most closely match your needs. Play around with varying pressure levels, stimulation durations, and patterns. For example, if your goal is to unwind before bed, think about combining deep breathing exercises with Shenmen (HT7) stimulation. If you want to work on physical discomfort, try kneading Zusanli (ST36) in a Shiatsu-style manner.

Recall that the secret is to strike a balance between making sure you're comfortable and successfully stimulating the spots. Adjust your technique gradually in accordance with your body's reaction and your changing sleep requirements.

Step4: Creating Your Schedule

Creating a customized acupressure practice entails combining your selected points and methods in a logical order. To center yourself, start your routine with a few minutes of deep breathing or meditation. Proceed to the acupressure points you have chosen, giving each enough time. Keep your awareness present and concentrate on the feelings you are experiencing as you stimulate the locations.

Think about arranging your daily schedule to include your acupressure routine. Consistency is essential, whether it's for a pre-bedtime routine, a noon stress-relieving session, or peaceful periods during wakeful nights.

Step 5: Change and Progress

Stay aware of your body's cues as you set out on your unique acupressure journey. Modify your regimen in accordance with your changing demands and sleep patterns. To monitor changes in the quality of your sleep, keep a sleep journal where you record the nights when your routine resulted in especially peaceful sleep and the times when you faced difficulties.

In the event that new pressures arise or your sleep patterns change, review and modify your routine. And don't be afraid to ask acupressure specialists or medical professionals for advice when necessary.

You may empower yourself to mindfully and intentionally navigate the complex world of sleep by creating a customized acupressure program. By interacting with this customized method, you develop a deep connection between traditional knowledge and contemporary requirements, ultimately accepting the acupressure's transformative power on your path to better sleep and overall health.

CHAPTER 6

Complementary Techniques for Better Sleep: Discuss other holistic approaches that can complement acupressure therapy, such as relaxation exercises, breathing techniques, and dietary adjustments to enhance the overall sleep-promoting effect.

When it comes to restoring sleep and conquering insomnia, a multimodal strategy that incorporates a range of holistic methods can be quite effective. Although acupressure therapy is a powerful tool for treating sleep disorders, its effectiveness can be increased by incorporating supplementary methods that promote overall wellbeing, balance, and relaxation. This section examines a number of these methods, such as breathing exercises, dietary changes, and relaxation exercises, which work in concert to provide a thorough and potent plan for improving sleep.

1. Meditation Activities

Relaxation exercises are a collection of techniques meant to ease mental and physical tension and prepare the body for sound sleep. People can relax and get ready for sleep with the use of methods including mindfulness meditation, progressive muscle relaxation, and guided imagery.

People who practice progressive muscle relaxation methodically tense and release different muscle groups, which facilitates physical relaxation and releases built-up stress. On the other side, guided imagery makes use of the power of visualization to conjure up peaceful mental images that help the mind relax. By promoting present-moment awareness, mindfulness meditation helps people let go of their daily concerns and cultivate a calm state of mind that promotes sleep.

2. Inhalation Methods

One essential component of human physiology that directly affects how the nervous system reacts to stress is breathing. Including particular breathing exercises in a nightly regimen can help the body transition into a more relaxed state and get ready for sleep.

For example, the 4-7-8 breathing technique calls for four counts of inhalation, seven counts of holding the breath, and eight counts of exhalation. Calm is induced by this pattern, which activates the parasympathetic nervous system. Similar to this, deep breathing from the diaphragm as opposed to shallow breathing from the chest can cause relaxation reactions and lessen anxiety.

3. Nutritional Modifications

The foods we eat during the day can have a big effect on how well we sleep. The choice of foods that promote sleep as well as the timing of meals are two dietary modifications that help improve sleep.

Sleep can be facilitated by eating foods high in tryptophan, an amino acid that is a precursor to melatonin and serotonin. Dairy products, nuts, seeds, and turkey are some examples of these foods. Low-glycemic carbohydrates, such as whole grains, also promote stable blood sugar levels, which helps to avoid sleep disturbances brought on by energy swings.

Additionally, eating with awareness and steering clear of large or spicy meals right before night might ease pain and facilitate simpler digestion. Limiting caffeine consumption can help keep its stimulating effects from disrupting the body's normal sleep-wake cycle, particularly in the later part of the day.

Technology Cleansing and Sleep Maintenance

The widespread use of electronics and exposure to blue light just before bed might interfere with the body's melatonin production, which makes it more difficult to fall asleep. Adopting proper sleep hygiene practices and starting a technology detox an hour or so before bedtime can greatly improve the quality of your sleep.

Maintaining a comfortable mattress and pillows, controlling the temperature in the room, and reducing light and noise disruptions are all important steps in creating a sleep-friendly atmosphere. Maintaining a regular sleep pattern, which involves going to bed and waking up at the same times every day, helps to improve sleep efficiency by supporting the body's internal clock.

5. Aromatherapy and Herbal Teas

Herbal teas with naturally relaxing qualities, such those made with chamomile, valerian root, and passionflower, can help induce relaxation and get the body ready for sleep. As part of your nightly ritual, you can sip these teas to help unwind and create a calming environment.

Aromatherapy is the use of essential oils to promote relaxation and mood. One herb that has been demonstrated to lower anxiety and enhance sleep quality is lavender. Aromatherapy, whether it be from diffusers or diluted essential oils, can be included into a pre-bed bath to produce a relaxing sensory experience.

Final Thoughts

Getting restorative sleep is a journey that involves more than one strategy. People can develop a comprehensive toolkit for improving their sleep by adopting alternative strategies such as breathing exercises, diet changes, technology detoxification, herbal therapies, and aromatherapy.

These methods complement acupressure therapy, enhancing its benefits and addressing various aspects of sleep problems. The combination of these holistic approaches provides a comprehensive solution that not only helps people overcome insomnia but also builds a long-lasting foundation for overall well-being, particularly in light of the ways in which the modern world continues to disrupt our sleep habits. People who adopt a holistic perspective on sleep can set off on a journey of deep recovery, enjoying increased energy and a restored sense of connectedness to the cycles of sleep.

CHAPTER 7

Lifestyle Factors and Sleep Hygiene: Highlight the importance of maintaining a healthy sleep environment and adopting proper sleep hygiene practices alongside acupressure therapy to achieve optimal results.

It is impossible to overstate the benefits of combining acupressure therapy with a comfortable sleeping environment in the quest for undisturbed sleep and restored health. This chapter explores the complex interplay between acupressure, sleep hygiene, and lifestyle factors, providing a thorough road map for achieving optimal sleep outcomes through harmonic integration.

The Ecology and Well-Being Dance

Think of your sleeping environment as the stage on which your sleep act takes place. As a dancer needs a comfortable and well-lit stage, so too do the surroundings you create affect the quality of your sleep. Although acupressure affects the body's internal energies, a comfortable sleeping environment offers the outside reinforcement required for those energies to thrive.

Building the Sleep Haven

Start by assessing your sleeping area. Is it a center of distractions or a haven of peace? Establish a sanctuary for rest by making sure of the following:

1. Tune Down the Lights: Man-made illumination throws off the body's circadian cycle. When going to bed, choose gentle, warm lighting to let your body know it's time to relax.

2. Comfort is Key: Make an investment in pillows and a

mattress that will accommodate your individual sleeping style. Take into account elements like material, breathability, and firmness.

3. Declutter and Destress: Remove all unnecessary items and distractions from your sleeping space. Set aside time for rest and sleep, keeping it apart from work or other mentally taxing pursuits.

4. Temperature Control: To promote the best possible sleep, keep your room at a comfortable temperature, usually between 65

and 72 degrees Fahrenheit (18 and 22 degrees Celsius).

5. Noise Reduction: If needed, use earplugs or white noise devices to reduce distracting noises. Make relaxing noises in your environment.

The Harmonious Practices of Sleep Hygiene

Similar to how a symphony is composed of different instruments, good sleep hygiene habits work in unison to improve the overall quality of your sleep. Acupressure can be used in conjunction with these techniques to increase their efficacy:

1. Regular Sleep Schedule: Establish a sleep routine that involves going to bed and waking up at the same times every day. This assists in balancing the internal clock of your body.

2. Screen Curfew: Minimize screen time at least one hour prior to going to bed. Device blue light can inhibit the creation of melatonin, which makes it difficult to fall asleep.

3. Mindful Eating and Hydration: Steer clear of large, heavy, or spicy meals right before bed. Remain hydrated, but cut back on liquids closer to bedtime to avoid morning headaches.

4. Physical Activity: Work out on a regular basis, but try to wrap up a few hours before night to give your body time to relax.

5. Stress Management: To help you cope with stress and worry, incorporate relaxation methods into your daily routine, such as

meditation, deep breathing, or mild yoga.

Acupressure and Environment: A Dancing Couple

When a comfortable sleeping environment is combined with acupressure, the results are a harmonious dance that maximizes the advantages of both practices. Arrange your sleeping space to promote calm and relaxation before engaging in acupressure. As you work on the acupoints, let your body and mind to synchronize with the calm environment you've created.

Additionally, the space where you sleep acts as a canvas for the healing effects of acupressure. Improved circulation, less tension, and a regulated energy flow work in concert with the outside factors that maximize the quality of sleep.

Final Thoughts

Acupressure therapy and a sleep-friendly setting combine to create a lovely symphony that harmonizes with your body's natural rhythms.

You may build a holistic approach to sleep enhancement by combining acupressure with good sleep hygiene and creating a peaceful sleep sanctuary. Combining age-old knowledge with contemporary living means that you will set out on a revolutionary path toward bright days and peaceful nights, taking into account the whole range of elements that go into creating your sleep symphony.

CHAPTER 8

**Success Stories and Testimonials:
Share real-life success stories and
testimonials from individuals
who have benefited from one
point acupressure for insomnia,
showcasing the transformative
impact it can have on their sleep
quality and overall well-being.**

The path to beating insomnia and getting good sleep is a very personal one that is frequently characterized by weariness, frustration, and a desperate search for answers. This chapter explores the incredible success stories and moving testimonies of people who have felt the life-changing effects of one-point acupressure for insomnia. These stories not only demonstrate the effectiveness of acupressure, but they also offer hope to anyone seeking to restore their general health and quality of sleep.

Jennifer's Path: Taking Back the Evening

In her late thirties, Jennifer was a busy worker who had struggled with terrible insomnia for many years. She would often have restless nights, which left her exhausted, agitated, and finding it difficult to concentrate during the day. Conventional drugs caused unwanted side effects and provided only patchy comfort.

Jennifer looked to acupressure therapy in a desperate attempt to find a natural remedy. She discovered the Anmian pressure point, which is located behind the ear and is well known for helping people sleep soundly. She added acupressure to her nighttime ritual despite her skepticism and willingness to try anything.

Within a few weeks, Jennifer started to notice a significant change. She felt peaceful as she pressed the Anmian point softly before going to bed. Her speeding mind finally calmed down to reveal a peaceful mental terrain. Sleep was taking hold of her more and more each night, and the once-unreal feeling of waking up feeling rejuvenated became her new normal.

Jennifer's experience is a perfect example of how acupressure may be used to break free from the snare of sleeplessness. The Anmian pressure point turned became her ally, a transformational touchpoint that led her into the domain of restorative sleep.

Mark's Narrative: From Restless Nights to Peace

Insomnia was an unwanted companion brought on by the horrors of battle experiences for Mark, a veteran of the military. He was emotionally and physically exhausted by the constant restlessness and terrible dreams that plagued his evenings. Traditional therapies only brought temporary relief, and Mark longed for a more all-encompassing strategy to help him sleep again.

Mark started focusing on the Shenmen pressure point on his earlobe after learning about acupressure from a friend. Mark found that this pressure point—which is linked to emotional equilibrium and serenity—became indispensable in his fight against sleeplessness. He experienced a change in his emotional terrain with each soft touch—a slow release of the weights he had been carrying for years.

Mark's nights became calmer and more orderly over time. The effect of the Shenmen pressure point on his emotional condition resulted in a resurgence of inner peace in addition to the relief of nightmares. As Mark's sleeplessness lifted, his days become easier to handle and he discovered that he had more energy to enjoy life.

Elena's Statement: Adopting a Holistic Approach to Healing

Three-time mother Elena had struggled with sleep disturbances ever since her youngest kid was born. She had little time to treat her insomnia, which showed up as trouble falling asleep and frequent awakenings, because of the responsibilities of being a parent. She chose to research the advantages of acupressure after learning about its potential.

Between her eyebrows is the Yintang pressure point, which served as the focal point of Elena's acupressure journey. A surge of calm washed through her as she gently pressed on this spot. Her mind started to clear of the constant concerns that had been bothering her, making it easier for her to fall asleep peacefully.

Elena's testimonial illustrates how acupressure works on a comprehensive level. Elena was able to access a healing potential that she could use in her day-to-day life as a mother and caregiver by addressing not just the physical but also the emotional and mental components of sleep.

A Transformative Tapestry

These testimonies and success stories create a tapestry of change that shows how one-point acupressure for insomnia may completely change people's life.

Jennifer, Mark, and Elena found that a single touchpoint can have a powerful impact that goes much beyond the tangible world. With its capacity to realign the nerve system, alleviate mental stress, and promote calmness, acupressure presents a comprehensive strategy for rest that strikes a deep chord with people.

These tales emphasize the value of individualized treatment plans as well. Since every person's path is different, acupressure allows for customisation, allowing people to find pressure spots that are in tune with their own needs.

Final Thoughts: A Slant on Hope

For those struggling with the grip of insomnia, the success stories and testimonies presented in this chapter offer hope. Readers are shown the transformational power of one-point acupressure for insomnia through the perspectives of Jennifer, Mark, and Elena. This technique is a beacon of hope that illuminates the path towards reviving sleep and restoring well-being.

These stories serve as a helpful reminder that the path to improved sleep is determined by more than just where you end up; it also depends on how brave you are to look into and accept holistic therapy options. The touch of acupressure turns into a language of self-care, softly pointing people in the direction of their well-deserved haven of rest. These tales demonstrate the ongoing ability of traditional methods to foster a strong bond between the body, mind, and sleep while also having a good impact on contemporary life.